# Remedy For Thyroid Problem

## Instant Thyroid and Hyperthyroidism healing strategies

By

## Dr. Elliott Charles

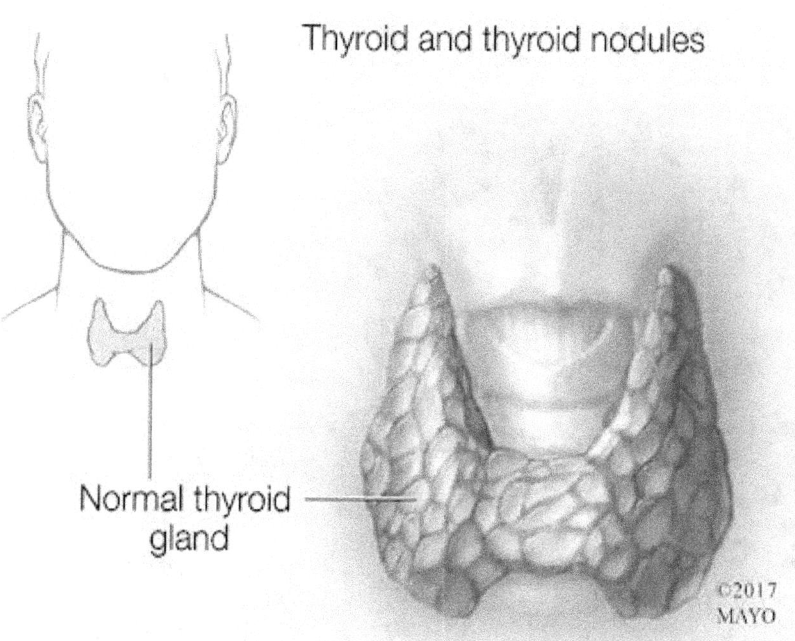


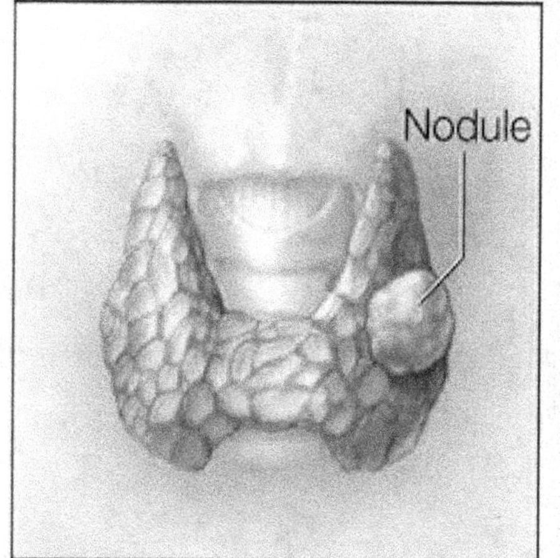


Thyroid with single nodule

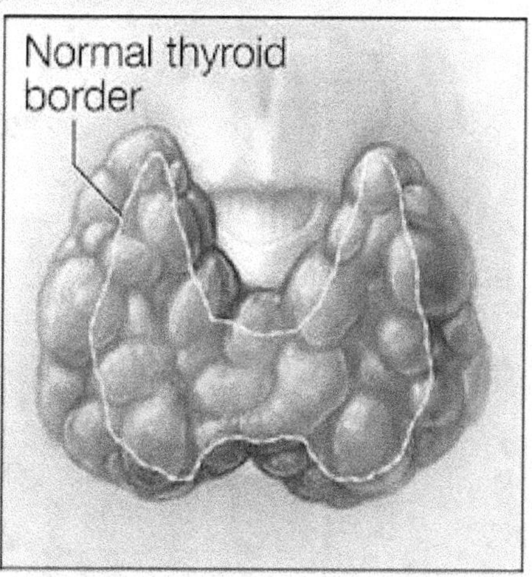


Thyroid with multiple nodules
(Multi-nodular goiter)

# 15 HEALING FOODS THAT ARE GOOD FOR YOUR THYROID

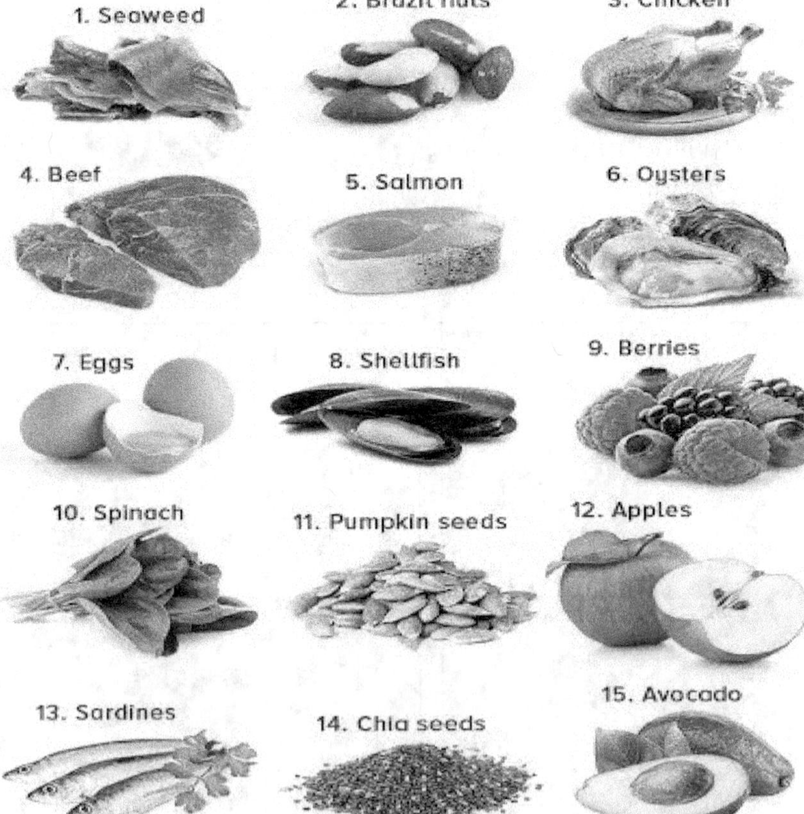

# Table Of Contents

# Introduction

the thyroid condition Your thyroid is responsible for the generation of hormones that regulate multiple body systems. When your thyroid produces too few or too many of these vital hormones, you get a thyroid condition. There are several different types of thyroid disease, including thyroiditis, hyperthyroidism, hypothyroidism, and Hashimoto's thyroiditis.

The thyroid gland is a small organ that is wrapped around the windpipe (trachea) in the front of the neck. It has two wide wings that wrap around the side of your throat and is the size of a butterfly in the middle. One gland is the thyroid. All over your body, there are glands that make and release substances that help your body do something. Your thyroid produces hormones that aid in controlling numerous body functions.

Your entire body can be affected when your thyroid doesn't work properly. Hyperthyroidism is a condition that can occur if your body produces an excessive amount of thyroid hormone. Hypothyroidism is a disorder in which your body generates insufficient thyroid hormone. Your healthcare provider must treat these two serious conditions.

Thyroid hormones, which regulate metabolism, are released and controlled by your thyroid, which plays a crucial role in your body. The process of converting food into energy is known as metabolism. This energy is used all throughout your body to maintain the proper functioning of numerous systems. Your metabolism is like a generator. It uses the energy it gets from the ground to power something much bigger.

T4 (thyroxine, which has four iodide atoms) and T3 (triiodothyronine, which has three iodine atoms) are two of the specific hormones that the thyroid produces to regulate metabolism. The thyroid makes these two hormones, which tell the body's cells how much energy to use. When your thyroid is functioning properly, it will keep the right amount of hormones in your body so that your metabolism runs at the right rate. The thyroid makes substitutes for the hormones as they are used up.

The pituitary gland, or something like it, is in charge of all of this. The pituitary gland, which is below your brain in the center of the skull, is responsible for monitoring and regulating the number of thyroid hormones in your bloodstream. The pituitary gland will adjust hormone levels with its own hormone if it detects a low or high level of thyroid hormones in your body. Thyroid-stimulating hormone (TSH) is the name of this hormone. The TSH will be delivered to the thyroid, where it will instruct the thyroid on how to restore normal function.

Thyroid disease is an umbrella term for a medical problem that prevents your thyroid from producing the appropriate amount of hormones. Typically, your thyroid produces hormones that keep your body working smoothly. When your thyroid produces too much thyroid hormone, your body burns through energy too quickly. This is known as hyperthyroidism. Consuming energy too quickly might cause your heart to beat quicker, causing you to lose weight without On the other hand, your thyroid may produce inadequate thyroid hormone. This is known as hypothyroidism. When you have insufficient thyroid hormone in your body, you may feel weary, gain weight, and be unable to endure cold temperatures.

These two primary diseases can be caused by a variety of factors. They can also be inherited (given down through families).

# Chapter one

# Knowing The Fundamentals Of Thyroid

Your thyroid is an essential endocrine gland that is responsible for the production and release of particular hormones. The primary function of your thyroid is to regulate your metabolism, or the way your body uses energy. Your thyroid may malfunction occasionally. These ailments are prevalent and treatable.

Describe the thyroid.
Observe World Rabies Day on Sept. 28 to help raise awareness about rabies and the importance of rabies prevention.
Under your skin, at the front of your neck, is the small, butterfly-shaped gland known as your

thyroid. It is a part of your endocrine system and produces and secretes certain hormones, which control many important body functions. The primary function of your thyroid is to regulate your metabolism (metabolic rate), which is the process by which your body converts food into energy. Your body's cells require energy to function.

Your entire body can be affected when your thyroid is not functioning properly.

**What is the endocrine system?**

The endocrine system: what is it?

The various glands that make and release hormones make up your endocrine system.

An organ that produces one or more substances, such as hormones, digestive fluids, sweat, or tears, is known as a gland. Hormones are released directly into the bloodstream by endocrine glands.

Hormones are substances that communicate with your organs, skin, muscles, and other tissues via your bloodstream in order to coordinate various body activities. These signals tell your body when and what to do.

Your endocrine system consists of the following glands and organs:

Hypothalamus.
the hypothalamus.
Thyroid.
Thyrotoxic glands.
The adrenal glands
gland of pineal.
Pancreas.
Ovaries.
Testes.

**Why does my thyroid function?**

As an endocrine organ, your thyroid makes and secretes chemicals. The following hormones are made and released by your thyroid:

T4 thyroxine: This is the primary hormone produced and released by your thyroid. Your metabolism is not significantly impacted by this hormone, even though your thyroid makes the most of it. Through a process known as deiodination, your thyroid can convert T4 into T3 once it has released it into your bloodstream.

T3: Triiodothyronine T3, which has a greater impact on metabolism than T4, is produced by your thyroid in smaller amounts than T4.

Triiodothyronine in reverse (RT3): Your thyroid makes tiny measures of RT3, which turns around the impacts of T3.

Calcitonin: Your blood calcium level is controlled by this hormone.

Your thyroid gland needs iodine, which can be found in food (most commonly iodized table salt) and water, to produce thyroid hormones. Iodine is converted into thyroid hormones by the thyroid gland. The amount of hormones produced and released by your thyroid can be affected by having too much or too little iodine in your body.

The following bodily functions are affected by your thyroid hormones:

how you use energy in your body (metabolism).

Heart rate

Breathing.

Digestion.

The temp of the body.

The growth of the brain.

Activity of the mind.

Preserving the skin and bones.

Fertility.

**What other glands and organs are involved in the thyroid's function?**

An intricate system of glands and hormones is your endocrine system. Many hormones and glands depend on signals from other hormones and glands to start working. Additionally, some hormones have the ability to inhibit other hormones.

Thyroid hormone levels are controlled by a complicated system in your body. To start with, your nerve center (a piece of your mind situated on the undersurface of it) secretes thyroid-delivering chemical (TRH), which invigorates a piece of your pituitary organ to emit thyroid-invigorating chemical (TSH). If your body has enough iodine, TSH causes your thyroid follicular cells to release thyroxine (T4) and triiodothyronine (T3).

Most of your body's organs and systems are influenced by your thyroid gland and its hormones, including:

Your circulatory system: The amount of blood that your heart pumps through your circulatory system (cardiac output), your heart rate, and the force and vigor with which your heart contracts (contractility of the heart) are all regulated by your thyroid.

Your system of nerves: When your thyroid isn't working as it should, it can cause numbness, tingling, pain, or a burning sensation in the areas of your body that are affected. Additionally, hypothyroidism and hyperthyroidism both have the potential to cause anxiety.

Your system of digestion: How food moves through your digestive system (gastrointestinal motility) is influenced by your thyroid.

Your genital organs: Infertility issues and irregular menstrual periods are both possible outcomes of a dysfunctional Thyroid.

**Is it possible to survive without a thyroid?**

It is possible to live without a thyroid. However, in order to maintain your health and avoid certain side effects and symptoms, you will need to take hormone replacement therapy for the rest of your life. A common procedure that can treat certain thyroid conditions is thyroid removal surgery, also known as a thyroidectomy.

**The thyroid is situated where?**

The trachea, or front of your neck, is where you'll find your thyroid gland. It resembles a butterfly in that it is smaller in the middle and has two wide wings that wrap around your throat. When you press your finger to the front of your neck, you can't feel a healthy thyroid gland because it is usually not visible from the outside (there is no lump on your neck).

**What are the parts of the thyroid?**
The thyroid is made up of two main parts: the middle of the thyroid, which connects the two halves (lobes), and the two halves (lobes).
Thyroid follicle cells (thyrocytes) and C-cells, which secrete the hormone calcitonin, make up your thyroid. Thyrocytes make and store thyroid hormone (mostly T3 and T4).

**How big is the thyroid?**
Your thyroid has a length of about 2 inches. You can't see a healthy thyroid by looking at your neck because it usually doesn't stick out of your throat.
However, your thyroid can become enlarged due to certain conditions. Goiter is the name for this. You might experience the following signs and symptoms if you have a goiter:
swelling just below the Adam's apple in the front of your neck.
a sensation of tightness around your throat.
a change in your voice, like hoarseness (a voice that is scratchy).

**What diseases and circumstances impact the thyroid?**

Thyroid disorders come in a variety of forms. An estimated 20 million people in the United States suffer from some kind of thyroid disorder, making it a very common condition. Thyroid disorders are diagnosed five to eight times more frequently in women and people assigned female at birth (AFAB) than in men and people assigned male at birth (AMAB).

Varieties of Thyroid Disease, both primary and secondary

Your thyroid gland is where primary thyroid disease begins. Your pituitary gland is where secondary thyroid disease begins. Primary hyperthyroidism, for instance, is characterized by a thyroid nodule releasing excessive amounts of thyroid hormones. Secondary hyperthyroidism occurs when a pituitary tumor releases excessive amounts of thyroid-stimulating hormone (TSH), which causes your thyroid to produce excessive amounts of thyroid hormones.

**The four main conditions that affect your thyroid**

Underactive thyroid or hypothyroidism

Hyperthyroidism (overactive thyroid).

Goiter is a thyroid condition.

Thyroid malignant growth.

Hypothyroidism An underactive thyroid, also known as hypothyroidism, occurs when your thyroid does not produce and release sufficient amounts of thyroid hormones. Your metabolism slows down in some ways as a result of this. It is a condition that affects approximately 10 million people in the United States and is fairly prevalent. It can be treate

An autoimmune condition known as Hashimoto's disease

Thyroiditis (thyroid inflammation)

Absence of iodine.

a thyroid gland that isn't working right (when the thyroid doesn't work right from birth).

medication overtreatment of hyperthyroidism.

Removal of the thyroid glands.

Overactive thyroid, also known as hyperthyroidism, is a condition in which your thyroid produces and releases more thyroid hormones than your body requires. Your metabolism picks up some parts as a result. In the United States, hyperthyroidism affects about one in every 100 people over the age of 12. It can be treated.

Hyperthyroidism can be caused by

Autoimmune disease Graves' disease

Thyroid knobs.

Thyroiditis (thyroid inflammation)

Thyroiditis postpartum (inflammation of the thyroid following childbirth)

excess iodine in your blood due to medication or diet.

medication overtreatment of hypothyroidism.

a pituitary gland tumor that is not malignant.

A goiter is a thyroid gland enlargement.. Goiters are fairly prevalent; Goiters have a variety of causes, depending on the type, and affect approximately 5% of Americans

Goiters have different causes, depending on their types

Simple goiters: When your thyroid gland doesn't make enough hormones to meet your body's needs, these goiters form. By expanding, your thyroid gland tries to make up for the lack.

Endothelial goiter: These goiters appear in people whose diet lacks iodine, which is necessary for the production of thyroid hormone. In the United States and a number of other nations, iodine is added to table salt, preventing endemic goiter inhabitant populations.

Goiters on occasion: Most of the time, these goiters have no known cause. Some medications, like lithium, can occasionally result in sporadic goiters.


Thyroid cancer

Cancer of the thyroid Cancer of the thyroid begins in the tissues of the thyroid gland. Thyroid cancer affects approximately 53,000 people in the United States annually. The majority of thyroid cancers respond well to treatment.

The type of cells from which cancer grows determines the classification of thyroid cancer. Types of thyroid cancer include:

Papillary: Papillary thyroid cancer accounts for up to 80% of all cases.

Follicular: Up to 15% of thyroid cancer diagnoses involve follicular thyroid cancer.

Medullary: Medullary thyroid cancer accounts for about 2% of cases. Frequently, a gene mutation is the cause.

Anaplastic: Anaplastic thyroid cancer accounts for about 2% of cases.

# Chapter Two

# Common techniques for assessing the thyroid's health?

A blood test that measures your levels of thyroid-stimulating hormone (TSH) is the first test used to check your thyroid's health. Both hypothyroidism and hyperthyroidism can be detected with this test.

A TSH blood test typically finds results between 0.5 and 5.0 mIU/L, or milli-international units per liter. However, this may differ from laboratory to laboratory and from person to person, as well as from age and pregnancy.
Your blood levels of the thyroid hormones T4 and T3 can also be checked by your doctor.

A thyroid ultrasound or thyroid scan, which uses small amounts of a safe, radioactive material to create images of your thyroid, may be suggested by your doctor if your test results are abnormal.

**What are the early indicators and signs of thyroid issues?**
The symptoms of various thyroid conditions differ. However, due to the fact that your thyroid plays a significant role in certain body systems and processes, including the regulation of temperature, metabolism, and heart rate, there are a few symptoms to look out for that could indicate a thyroid condition:

Heart rate that is either sluggish or rapid.
Weight gain or loss that is unexplainable.

difficulty coping with heat or cold.

Anxiety or sadness

Periods that don't come on time.

A blood test to check your thyroid function should be discussed with your healthcare provider if you are experiencing any of these symptoms.

**Treatments for thyroid issues**

The thyroid is prevented from producing hormones by these drugs. This may be prescribed by healthcare providers for hyperthyroidism.

Beta-blockers: These medications help treat hyperthyroidism's symptoms, like a fast heartbeat, but they don't treat the condition of the thyroid.

Iodine radioactive: Your thyroid gland will eventually be destroyed as a result of this medication's damage to thyroid cells. Thyroid cancer and hyperthyroidism can both be treated with this.

Medication for thyroid hormone: Hypothyroidism can be treated with these medications, which are synthetic versions of thyroid hormones. Most of the time, people who have a thyroidectomy or have a thyroid that doesn't work because of radioactive iodine need to take these medications for the rest of their lives.

Surgery

Thyroidectomy is the type of surgery that is most frequently associated with thyroid conditions. The surgical removal of your entire thyroid gland is known as a thyroidectomy. Thyroidectomy is the first-line treatment for thyroid cancer and one of the treatments for thyroid disease.

A lobectomy, in which only a portion of your thyroid is removed, is another option for surgery.

**Radiation therapy and chemotherapy**

Thyroid cancer can be treated with radiation therapy or chemotherapy. Both treatments stop cancer cells from growing and killing them. Radiation or chemotherapy are not necessary for the majority of thyroid cancer cases.

**What factors increase the likelihood of developing a thyroid condition?**

Thyroid disorders are prevalent and can affect people of any age. However, the following factors increase your risk of developing a thyroid condition:

having a history of thyroid disease in the family.

having an autoimmune disease, such as lupus, rheumatoid arthritis, or type 1 diabetes.

taking medication with a lot of iodine in it.

Being over the age of 60, particularly if you are a woman or someone whose gender was chosen at birth (AFAB).

**How can I maintain a healthy thyroid?**
Making sure your diet contains enough iodine is the most important thing you can do to keep your thyroid healthy. To produce thyroid hormones, your thyroid requires iodine. The good news is that foods fortified with iodine and iodized table salt provide the majority of people with sufficient amounts of iodine.

Food sources that contain iodine
Cheese.
Milk from cows
Eggs.
Yogurt.
Fish from the sea.
Shellfish.
Seaweed.
Soy milk.
sour cream.

However, it is essential to avoid overconsuming iodine due to its potential negative effects. Don't be afraid to talk to your doctor if you have any questions or concerns about your thyroid health.

When should I see my thyroid specialist?
Contact your doctor right away if you notice changes in your weight, heart rate, or sensitivity to temperature as signs of thyroid disease. To determine if your symptoms are caused by your thyroid, they can conduct a straightforward blood test.
Your thyroid is a crucial part of your endocrine system that controls many body functions. Thyroid disorders are extremely prevalent and treatable. Don't be afraid to talk to your doctor if you have any symptoms of thyroid disease or want to know if you have any risk factors for developing thyroid disease. They are prepared to assist you.

# Chapter Three

# Understanding How Hyperthyroidism Affects the Thyroid

Hyperthyroidism is the condition in which your thyroid gland produces too many thyroid hormones. This may result in symptoms such as decreased appetite and weight loss.

**Why does hyperthyroidism occur?**
Hyperthyroidism can be caused by a number of conditions, the most common of which is Graves' disease.

The thyroid is a small gland in the front of your neck that looks like a butterfly. Thyroxine (T4) and triiodothyronine (T3), the two main hormones that control how your cells use energy, are produced by it. Through the release of these hormones, your metabolism is controlled by your thyroid gland.

When your thyroid produces an excessive amount of T3, T4, or both, it speeds up your body's systems, which can be distressing. Symptoms can be alleviated and complications can be avoided if hyperthyroidism is diagnosed and treated promptly.

**What is the root of hyperthyroidism?**
Hyperthyroidism can be caused by a variety of conditions. Graves' disease, an autoimmune illness, is the most prevalent cause of hyperthyroidism. In Graves' disease, antibodies from your immune system attack your thyroid gland, causing too much hormone to be releasedTrusted Source.
Females are more likely than males to develop Graves' disease. According to an overview of a 2011 study by Trusted Source, genetics play a major role in determining whether a person will develop Graves' disease, but environmental factors also play a role. Graves' disease is not caused by a single gene defect but rather by minor changes in multiple genes, according to family and twin studies.
So that they can accurately assess your risk factors, tell your doctor about any relatives who have been diagnosed with hyperthyroidism.

Other causes of hyperthyroidism, in addition to Graves' disease

Too much iodine. Iodine, which is a key component of T4 and T3, can temporarily cause hyperthyroidism if consumed in excessive amounts. Iodine can be absorbed through dairy products and fish. Cough syrups, amiodarone (a medicine used to treat heart arrhythmia), and medical contrast dyes all contain it.

Thyroiditis (thyroid inflammation) Thyroiditis is a condition in which the thyroid gland swells and produces excessive or inadequate amounts of the hormone.

benign tumors on the thyroid The term "nodules" refers to lumps that form on the thyroid gland, typically for unknown reasons. A few thyroid knobs produce overabundance thyroid chemicals, yet the greater part are harmless. Adenoma and benign tumor are other names for nodules.

Thyroid nodules that are harmful Malignant nodules on the thyroid can cause cancer. A type of tissue biopsy known as fine needle aspiration or ultrasoundTrusted Source can be used to determine whether a nodule is benign or malignant.

Testicular or ovarian tumors.

Blood with a lot of T4 in it. Taking certain dietary supplements or taking too much of the thyroid hormone medication levothyroxine can raise T4 levels.

Vs. Thyrotoxicosis

Vs. Hyperthyroidism and thyrotoxicosis are not the same thing, despite the fact that they are sometimes used interchangeably. In reality, all forms of hyperthyroidism fall under the category of thyrotoxicosis.

Your thyroid's physical overproduction of hormones is called hyperthyroidism. Thyrotoxicosis is the more general term for having too much thyroid hormone in your body, whether it came from the gland, a medication, or another source.

**Which signs and symptoms indicate hyperthyroidism?**

Some hyperthyroidism symptoms may be physically obvious, while others may be subtle and difficult to recognize at first. Anxiety is frequently mistaken for hyperthyroidism.

The following are typical signs and symptoms of hyperthyroidism, as stated by the National Institutes of Health (NIH) Trusted Source:

The thyroid gland itself can swell into a goiter, which can be symmetrical or one-sided. The symptoms of a goiter include weight loss but also an increased appetite, rapid or irregular heartbeat, nervousness, or irritability, fatigue, and difficulty sleeping. The symptoms of a goiter can also include hand tremors, muscle weakness, and becoming easily overheated. A goiter is an enlargement of the gland, and it typically appears as a lump or puffiness at the neck's base. Iodine deficiency is the most common cause of goiters, according to Trusted Source.

Eye protrusion or prominence is another possibility. Exophthalmos is the medical term for this, and it is linked to Graves' disease.

Brittle hair and hair loss can also result from untreated thyroid disease over time.

Hyperthyroidism can cause a person to lose consciousness, have trouble breathing, or have an irregular heartbeat. These symptoms necessitate prompt medical attention. Complications If left untreated, hyperthyroidism can increase the risk of:

Stormy thyroid Untreated hyperthyroidism can lead to a rare health condition known as a thyroid storm. When there are too many thyroid hormones in your body, it goes into overdrive. A thyroid storm is characterized by a fever, high blood pressure, and rapid heart rate, all of which have the potential to cause death.

Complications

Complications of pregnancy This includes pregnant women who develop hyperthyroidism and people who already have thyroid disorders. Pregnant women and their unborn children can be harmed by high levels of thyroid hormone. According to a trusted source, risks include miscarriage and premature birth. During pregnancy, regular thyroid hormone tests can reveal irregularities, and your doctor may recommend medication.

Osteoporosis. Osteoporosis is a condition in which your bones become brittle and thin as a result of hyperthyroidism. Bone health can be improved by taking calcium and vitamin D supplements during and after treatment. Osteoporosis can also be avoided by engaging in regular According to a study, thyroid cancer in hyperthyroid people is more "aggressive" and has a worse prognosis than in euthyroid patients (those with a healthy thyroid). overview of a 2018 study from Trusted Source.

Atrial fibrillation, a dangerous arrhythmia (irregular heartbeat) that can result in stroke and congestive heart failure, can also be caused by hyperthyroidism. Thyroid disorders can lead to serious health problems and even medical emergencies if left untreated. The majority of blood tests that are used to diagnose hyperthyroidism and other thyroid conditions are simple. If you think you might be experiencing signs of hyperthyroidism, see a doctor right away.

**How do medical professionals identify hyperthyroidism?**
A physical examination and the collection of your personal and family medical history are part of a doctor's evaluation for hyperthyroidism. Typically, hyperthyroidism is diagnosed by a doctor based on symptoms, clinical signs, and laboratory tests.

**Trusted Source's diagnostic tests**
Tests at the T4, free T4, and T3 levels. These tests determine the level of thyroid hormone (T4 and T3) in your blood. Test for the level of thyroid-stimulating hormone (TSH). TSH is a hormone produced by the pituitary gland that causes the

thyroid gland to produce hormones. Your pituitary gland responds to high levels of thyroid hormone by producing less TSH. A rapid onset of hyperthyroidism can be indicated by an abnormally low TSH.

Radioactive iodine uptake scan of the thyroid By measuring how much iodine your thyroid "takes up" from your bloodstream, this helps your doctor determine whether your thyroid is overactive. You will receive a small tablet or liquid containing iodine from your doctor. After that, a special camera will take pictures of your thyroid while you lie on a table. A thyroid scan, in particular, can determine whether the issue is affecting the entire gland or just one area.

Thyroid ultrasound. The size of the thyroid gland as a whole and any masses on or within it (such as nodules) can be measured with ultrasounds. An ultrasound can also be used by doctors to determine whether a mass is cystic or solid.

MRI or CT scans. A pituitary tumor can be detected with a CT or MRI.

While some of these tests can be ordered by primary care physicians, an endocrinologist is the best option.

**Medical treatment for hyperthyroidism**

How to treat hyperthyroidism with medication Anti-thyroid medications stop the thyroid from making hormones is the area of expertise of endocrinologists in the treatment and management of hormone-related health conditions. The most widely recognized enemy of thyroid prescriptions are a class called thionamides, which incorporates the medications methimazole (MMI) and propylthiouracil (PTU).

For decades, thionamides have been used to treat hyperthyroidism. They are considered safe for both children and adults, including pregnant womenTrusted Source. Inconvenient side effects of antithyroid medications include joint pain, hair loss, and a rash. They may damage the liver in rare instances.

If you're pregnant or planning to become pregnant, as well as if you take any other medications, tell your doctor. Always follow your doctor's prescriptions for medication.

Radioactive iodine
Radioactive iodine, or just "radioiodine," effectively kills the cells that make thyroid hormones without

harming other parts of the body. Typically, it is taken orally as a tablet or liquid.

The opposite condition, hypothyroidism, occurs in the majority of people who receive radioiodine treatment for hyperthyroidism. You will, however, take a thyroid hormone supplement on a daily basis because this is easier to treat. Thyroid cancer is also treated with higher doses of RAI.

RAI has been linked, in rare instances, to an increased risk of certain cancers when administered in sustained higher doses. In lower doses used to treat hyperthyroidism, this has not been demonstrated to be the case.

RAI treatment can have side effects, Trusted Source, especially at higher doses. Dry mouth, nausea, and neck pain are some of these. Fertility can also be affected by high doses of RAI treatment.

Risk factors

Risk factors In summary, the most significant risk factors for hyperthyroidism are as follows:

Sex. Hyperthyroidism is more common in females than in males. Experts believe that hormones could be to blame for this.

Pregnancy. In some people, pregnancy can cause hyperthyroidism, which can have negative effects on both the mother and the unborn child.

Age. Hyperthyroidism is thought to be more common in older people, especially after the age of 60.

Genetics. Usually, hyperthyroidism is more likely to develop if there is a history of it in the family.

exposure to iodine. You might get an excess of iodine from specific drugs or food sources.

having a different health issue. Pernicious anemia, primary adrenal insufficiency, and type 1 diabetes are thought to increase risk.

Reduce your hyperthyroidism risk factors by changing your lifestyle. This means getting enough exercise throughout the week, taking nutritional supplements if necessary, and eating a well-balanced diet. Make a plan with your doctor that includes your own goals.

Smoking has been found to increase your risk of Graves' disease in particular, so avoid it or try to quit. According to a large-scale Norwegian study from 2007, Trusted Source, smokers had higher levels of thyroid hormone than nonsmokers. Women who reported never smoking had a prevalence of hyperthyroidism that was approximately twice as high as that of current smokers.

Outlook

Your thyroid might start producing too much thyroid hormone for a number of different reasons. Hyperthyroidism can be brought on by having too much iodine in your body, being pregnant, or having a genetic predisposition to thyroid conditions like Graves' disease. Good nutrition, regular exercise, and quitting smoking can all help lower your risk.

Symptoms, blood tests, and imaging are used to diagnose hyperthyroidism. Medication, radioiodine therapy, and, if necessary, surgery to remove all or part of the thyroid gland are the primary treatments for this condition.

The cause of hyperthyroidism determines the condition's long-term outlook. Without treatment, most cases, including Graves' disease, will get worse and can even be fatal. The good news is that hyperthyroidism can be easily treated, and many people who have it can return to full health.

If you think you have health issues related to your thyroid, talk to your doctor. Goiter, severe fatigue, and unplanned weight loss are all common signs of hyperthyroidism. You might be referred to an endocrinologist, who will look at you and do the tests that are needed.

Contrasting hypo- and hyperthyroidism
**What is the distinction?**
Have you recently received a diagnosis of hypothyroidism? If so, you probably already know that your thyroid gland isn't working as well as it could. Additionally, some of the associated symptoms, such as tiredness, constipation, and forgetfulness, are probably all too familiar to you. It's frustrating to have these symptoms. But they can be managed with the right treatment plan.

**What exactly is hypothyroidism?**
Simply put, your thyroid gland does not produce enough hormones for optimal function. Every aspect of your body's metabolism is controlled by the thyroid gland. The gland's hormone production slows down in hypothyroidism. Your metabolism slows as a result, which can result in weight gain. About 4.6% of Americans suffer from hypothyroidism, which is a common condition.

The American Thyroid Association asserts that hypothyroidism cannot be treated. However, the disease can be treated with medications. The medication aims to restore hormone levels, improve thyroid function, and enable you to lead a normal life.

Hashimoto's thyroiditis is the most prevalent cause of hypothyroidism. Your body attacks its own immune system when you have this condition. Hypothyroidism develops as a result of the thyroid's inability to produce hormones as it should over time as a result of this attack. Hashimoto's thyroiditis, like many other autoimmune conditions, is more common in women than in men.

Hyperthyroidism

As its name suggests, hyperthyroidism occurs when your body becomes overactive and produces an excessive amount of the thyroid hormones thyroxine (T4) and triiodothyronine (T3). A rapid heartbeat, increased appetite, anxiety, heat sensitivity, and sudden weight loss are all symptoms of hyperthyroidism.

**Most common causes of hyperthyroidism Disease**

thyroiditis, or an inflammation of the thyroid, a thyroid nodule that produces too much T4 hormone, Graves' disease, which is an autoimmune condition, and hyperthyroidism, in which an irritation of the thyroid, called thyroiditis, allows too much thyroid hormone to enter the blood. This may cause discomfort and pain. Pregnancy has also been linked to thyroiditis. Usually, this is only temporary.

In both hypothyroidism and hyperthyroidism, thyroid nodules are common. These nodules are usually not harmful. These nodules can cause your thyroid to grow in size or produce too much T4 thyroid hormone in hyperthyroidism. Sometimes, doctors don't know why this happens.

The body attacks itself due to Graves' disease. The thyroid gland is able to produce too much thyroid hormone as a result of this attack. Hyperthyroidism is frequently caused by this autoimmune disease. Your thyroid produces too much thyroid hormone when you have Graves' disease.

Medication, radioactive iodine, or surgery can all be used to treat hyperthyroidism. Hyperthyroidism can lead to bone loss and irregular heartbeat if left untreated. Graves' disease and Hashimoto's thyroiditis can run in families.

**The distinctions between hypothyroidism and hyperthyroidism's symptoms**

The symptoms of hypothyroidism include tiredness, weight gain, and a slowed metabolism. Hyperthyroidism is the opposite. Your body's functions may slow down or stop altogether if your thyroid is underactive.

If you have hyperthyroidism, you might have more energy as opposed to less. You might lose weight rather than gain weight. You might also experience anxiety rather than depression.

Hormone levels are the most common difference between the two diseases. Hypothyroidism causes a reduction in hormone levels. Hyperthyroidism causes an increase in hormone production.

In the United States, hypothyroidism is more common than hyperthyroidism. However, it is not uncommon to have either an overactive or underactive thyroid. An important part of your treatment plan is finding a skilled doctor who focuses on the thyroid, typically an endocrinologist.

In addition to avoiding the aforementioned foods, it is essential to avoid additional iodine.

# Chapter Four

# How to Naturally Manage Thyroid and Hyperthyroidism

Even if it isn't mentioned on the label, herbal supplements can contain iodine. Keep in mind that even if you can buy a supplement over the counter, it may still be harmful to your body.
Consult a doctor before taking any supplements.
Iodine needs to be in balance for it to work. Iodine deficiency can result in hypothyroidism, whereas excessive iodine intake can cause hyperthyroidism.
Unless your doctor tells you to, do not take any iodine medication.

L-carnitine

L-carnitine is a natural supplement that can help treat hyperthyroidism.

L-carnitine is an amino acid derivative that occurs naturally in the body. Supplements for weight loss frequently contain it.

Additionally, it can be found in dairy products, fish, and meat. Here, you can learn about the advantages of L-carnitine.

Thyroid hormones are prevented from entering certain cells by carnitine. According to a 2001 study, the symptoms of hyperthyroidism, such as heart palpitations, tremors, and fatigue, can be reversed or prevented with L-carnitine.

Even though this research looks promising, there aren't enough studies to know for sure if L-carnitine is a good way to treat hyperthyroidism.

Historically, the plant bugleweed has been used to treat lung and heart conditions.

Bugleweed

According to a few different sources, bugleweed is a thyro suppressant, which means that it makes the thyroid gland work less well.

Unfortunately, there is insufficient data to determine whether it is an effective hyperthyroidism treatment. If you decide to take a herbal supplement like bugleweed, follow the manufacturer's instructions for how much to take and how often to take it, and consult your doctor before starting anything new.

 B-complex or B-12
If you have hyperthyroidism, you might also have a deficiency in vitamin B-12. A lack of vitamin B-12 can make you feel tired, weak, and dizzy.
A vitamin B-12 injection or supplement may be recommended by your doctor if you have a vitamin B-12 deficiency.
Although taking vitamin B-12 supplements can alleviate some of these symptoms, they cannot treat hyperthyroidism on their own.
Although you can buy B-12 and B-complex vitamins over-the-counter, you should always consult your doctor before taking any new supplements.

Selenium
According to a Trusted Source of research, selenium may be able to alleviate hyperthyroidism symptoms.

Selenium is a naturally occurring mineral that can be found in grains, nuts, beef, fish, soil, and water It can also be considered as an addition.

Thyroid eye disease (TED), which can be treated with selenium, is linked to Graves' disease, the most common cause of hyperthyroidism. However, keep in mind that TED is not present in everyone with hyperthyroidism.

According to other studies, hyperthyroidism cannot be treated with selenium alone. The research is still mixed in general, Trusted Source.

Selenium supplements should always be discussed with your physician due to the possibility of adverse effects and the fact that they should not be taken in conjunction with certain medications.

Lemon balm

It is thought that lemon balm, a plant in the mint family, can treat Graves' disease. This could be because it lowers the hormone that stimulates the thyroid (TSH).

Nevertheless, there is a dearth of research on this assertion. There's lacking proof to survey whether lemon ointment successfully treats hyperthyroidism.

Lemon balm can be taken in the form of a tea or as a supplement. As a stress management strategy, sitting down with a cup of lemon balm tea may at least be healing.

Essential oils of lavender and sandalwood Despite the widespread belief that essential oils can alleviate hyperthyroidism symptoms, little research has been conducted on this claimTS

Lavender and sandalwood essential oils
The essential oils of lavender and sandalwood, for instance, can help you feel more at ease and less anxious. This may assist you in combating hyperthyroidism-related anxiety and insomnia.

Glucomannan
Glucomannan is a dietary fiber that comes in the form of capsules, powders, and tablets. Aside from that, there isn't enough research to suggest that essential oils could help. It frequently comes from the konjac plant's root.

A promising 2007 Trusted Source study suggests that people with hyperthyroidism could use glucomannan to lower their thyroid hormone levels, but more research is needed.

Bonus

Hyperthyroidism typically necessitates professional medical care and monitoring.

Natural treatments can help you manage your symptoms but cannot take the place of thyroid medication.

Self-care, exercise, healthy eating, and stress management can all help. Thyroid function can return to normal with medication and a healthy lifestyle.

**Tips On How to Prevent Thyroid Disease**

According to the American Thyroid Association (ATA), more than 12% of the US population will develop a thyroid condition at some point in their lives. The fact that they have thyroid issues makes around 20 million Americans have a thyroid infection right now, and upwards of 60% of individuals uninformed. We've already talked about how this disease's symptoms typically show up in older people, making it hard to link them to the disease.

However, this does not make the disease any less troubling; rather, you must make every effort to effectively reduce your risk of the cardiovascular issues that typically accompany it by preventing it.

**Strategies on you can prevent thyroid disease**

Stop smoking if you're a smoker. Not only does this lower your risk of developing thyroid disease, but it also prevents a wide range of other health problems, including cardiovascular ones.

Cut back on soy. Although the popular ingredient is not necessarily harmful, it is contentious, particularly when thyroid health is taken into consideration.

During your x-rays, you should request a thyroid collar to shield your thyroid gland from radiation.

Take a look at selenium supplements. Selenium is a nutrient that helps your thyroid gland stay healthy. It is found in some proteins. You are already taking in enough selenium if you eat a healthy diet. In any case, you might think about expanding your selenium admission to support your resistant framework and abatement side effects of hypothyroidism.

Regularly see your doctor. Both your thyroid health and overall health benefit from regular checkups.

**Thyroid Disease Treatment Options**

Treatment Options for Thyroid Disease There are two distinct treatment options for thyroid disease, which can manifest as hypothyroidism or hyperthyroidism.

Keep in mind that thyroid disease is a condition that lasts a lifetime; however, with careful treatment, a person can still lead a normal and healthy life.

Levothyroxine, a synthetic hormone that boosts your thyroid's production, can be used to treat hypothyroidism, which is more common.

Hyperthyroidism is uncommon and harder to treat. Radiotherapy may be required to disable the gland and requires careful drug therapy to prevent excessive hormone production. Thyroid surgery is sometimes necessary.

Regardless of the type of thyroid disease you have, you will discuss treatment options with your doctor, who will choose the best course of action for you.

Chapter 5

**Reduced Risks of Thyroid and Hyperthyroidism in the Future**

There is nothing you can do to guarantee that you will not develop thyroid disease, but you can make choices that will reduce your risk. Up to 60% of the 20 million Americans who have the disease may not be aware of it.

This this section talks about a portion of the manners in which you can decrease your gamble of creating thyroid illness.

Ask for a Thyroid Collar for X-Rays

 If you are going to have an X-ray, request a thyroid collar. This is critical in particular for:

Dental X-rays X-rays of the spine, head, neck, or chest A thyroid collar resembles a turtleneck sweater's neck. It weighs a lot and is lined with lead. The most vulnerable part of your head and neck is your thyroid. Your thyroid gland is shielded from radiation exposure by the collar, which can cause thyroid cancer.

Stop Smoking Cigarette smoke: Toxins in cigarette smoke can harm your thyroid. Thiocyanate is one of these. Iodine uptake is disrupted by this substance, which may prevent thyroid hormone production.

The thyroid hormone thyroxine (T4) can generally rise as a result of smoking. Thyroid-stimulating hormone (TSH) levels may also be slightly reduced as a result. TSH directs your thyroid to produce hormones.

Smokers are more likely to develop Graves' disease, according to research. Hyperthyroidism, also known as overactive thyroid, is frequently brought on by this condition. Graves' orbitopathy, a Graves' disease-related eye condition caused by smoking, is another possibility. Quitting smoking is difficult. Consult your physician about treatment options that may assist you in quitting.

Do a Thyroid Neck

A thyroid neck check is one way to find a thyroid problem. Do a Thyroid Neck Check If the swelling and lumps are close to the surface, this simple test can identify them. However, keep in mind that many nodules cannot be felt or seen. See your doctor if you experience additional symptoms.

This straightforward screening can be performed in front of a mirror at home. Be certain to complete each step. If you detect anything out of the norm, consult your doctor.

Ease Up on Soy

Reduce Your Consumption of Soy You may be aware that eating too much soy can be detrimental to thyroid health. However late examination recommends eating soy is by and large protected, it is most likely best to do as such in moderation.

The vast majority with thyroid sickness take the thyroid chemical substitution levothyroxine. It is preferable to take this medication without food. Consume within 30 to 60 minutes.

Because soy can hinder your body's ability to absorb levothyroxine, you should wait until it has been four hours since you took your medication before eating it.

Get Celiac Disease Diagnosed and Treated

Celiac disease is an autoimmune condition that causes your intestines to react abnormally to gluten. Get Celiac Disease Diagnosed and Treated Wheat, rye, barley, oats, and other related grains all contain the protein gluten.

It is unclear why people with autoimmune thyroid conditions like Hashimoto's thyroiditis and Graves' disease are three times more likely to have celiac disease. The genetic component of autoimmune diseases may play a role. Additionally, both conditions are fairly common. Additionally, celiac disease hinders

See Your Healthcare Provider Regularly
with the absorption of vital minerals like selenium and iodine, which can lead to thyroid dysfunction.

Talk to your doctor if you think you might have celiac disease or be sensitive to gluten.

A significant dietary change is avoiding or limiting gluten. It is essential to only make changes of this kind under the direction of a healthcare professional. Visit Your Primary Care Physician on a Regular Basis Regular visits to your primary care physician are essential. If you are at risk of developing thyroid disease, this is especially true. For instance, if you have Graves' disease or Hashimoto's thyroiditis in your family, your doctor may want to check your thyroid hormone levels once a year.

At some point in their lives, a thyroid condition will affect more than 12% of people living in the United States. There is nothing you can do to guarantee that you will not develop thyroid disease, but you can make choices that will reduce your risk. Up to 60% of the 20 million Americans who have the disease may not be aware of it.

You can take steps to lower your risk of developing thyroid disease in this book

## 5 Common Misconceptions About Thyroid Disease

Ask for a Thyroid Collar for X-Rays to Lower Your Risk of Thyroid Disease Verywell / Cindy Chung If you are scheduled for an X-ray, you should request a thyroid collar. This is critical in particular for:

Dental X-rays
X-rays of the spine, head, neck, or chest A thyroid collar resembles a turtleneck sweater's neck. It weighs a lot and is lined with lead.
The most vulnerable part of your head and neck is your thyroid. Talk to your doctor about taking selenium supplements because selenium is a nutrient that can be found in some proteins. The collar shields your thyroid gland from radiation exposure, which can cause thyroid cancer.

Selenium
Selenium levels are highest in the adult body in the thyroid. Getting enough of this nutrient can help you prevent thyroid disease.

**What is Selenium and How Does It Work?**
Getting enough selenium during pregnancy can lower your risk of developing postpartum thyroiditis, which is a condition in which your thyroid becomes inflamed after your baby is born.
However, keep in mind that selenium-rich soil in the United States is abundant, and the majority of

people consume the recommended amount of selenium. Before starting selenium supplements, talk to your doctor.

Before taking selenium, talk to your doctor. Its function in thyroid health is still poorly understood.

Consider Fluoride's Role

Some studies suggest that people who live in areas where drinking water is fluoridated are more likely to develop hypothyroidism. In fact, studies suggest that high selenium levels may be a risk factor for developing type 2 diabetes.

This has not been found in other studies. Avoiding fluoride is generally not recommended until this connection is established.

If you are concerned about the health effects of fluoride, you should talk to your doctor about it.

Look Out for Perchlorates

Keep an eye out for perchlorates Perchlorates are salts that have no odor and no color. They naturally occur in some parts of the United States and dissolve in water. They are also made for rocket motors, fireworks, and explosives. They can be found in the water supply in some parts of the country.

Water contaminated with perchlorate is used to irrigate a lot of produce in the United States. This indicates that the food supply in the United States contains perchlorate, and many Americans are exposed to low levels.

Your thyroid produces thyroid hormones with iodine. Perchlorates can prevent your thyroid from absorbing iodine if you have high levels. It's a good idea to stay up to date on perchlorate contamination in your area and the safe drinking water levels for perchlorates. Consider having the well water tested for perchlorate contamination if you use it.

Keep Potassium Iodide on Hand

Potassium iodide, or KI, can be purchased over the counter. It might be useful to have in your family's emergency kit. In the unlikely event of a nuclear accident or an attack on a nuclear facility, it may be helpful. However, KI will not be helpful if you are not in the path of a radioactive plume.

Iodine is what your thyroid needs to work. This typically comes from your blood. However, it is unable to distinguish between radioactive iodine and regular iodine. The kind that is released from nuclear power plants or from radioactive materials during nuclear explosions is called radioactive iodine.

Thyroid cancer risk can be reduced by taking KI within the first few hours of exposure to radioactive iodine.

Your risk of developing thyroid cancer can be increased by exposure to radioactive iodine. It poses a particular threat to infants, young children, and the unborn. In order to prevent your thyroid from absorbing radioactive iodine, you take KI to saturate it with iodine12. However, there are some risks associated with taking KI. The benefits are thought to outweigh the risks in a radiation emergency.

Taking KI can lead to a variety of health issues Hypothyroidism and hyperthyroidism can be sparked or exacerbated by it.

It may make existing thyroid problems worse.

Conditions like the Jod-Basedow phenomenon and the Wolff-Chaikoff effect can result from it.

The salivary gland may become inflamed as a result.

Allergic reactions, gastrointestinal disturbances, and rashes are all possible side effects.

There are a number of reasons why you should only administer KI when local health authorities instruct you to do so during a nuclear emergency13.

Radioactive iodine isn't present in every radioactive release. If you need to take KI, only health professionals will know.

You can find out who needs to take KI, when to take it, how much to take, and how long to take it from the authorities.

There is very little chance that you will need to take KI if you are not in close proximity to a nuclear accident or release.

Preventing Hypothyroidism

When it comes to preventing hypothyroidism, most people can't do much to stop it from happening.

Iodine deficiency is prevalent in some nations, particularly in Africa and Southeast Asia. Iodized salt has been used in many countries to combat iodine deficiency. However, taking iodine supplements may aid in the prevention of hypothyroidism in nations where either salt is not commonly consumed or the element is not added to salt.

However, the majority of diets in developed nations, like the United States, contain sufficient amounts of iodine. However, even if you get enough iodine, there is no known way to prevent hypothyroidism.

Fortunately, hypothyroidism can be prevented from becoming serious. You can avoid serious complications that can occur if hypothyroidism is not treated by comprehending the risk factors, recognizing your symptoms, and receiving a diagnosis early on.

## What To Do for a Healthy Thyroid

The  conditions can result in issues with weight, digestion, and tiredness1. However, you might not think about your thyroid if it isn't causing you any problems.

Your thyroid's health may improve if you make a few changes to your diet and lifestyle.

## Going Mediterranean

Eating a well-balanced diet is one of the most important things you can do to keep your thyroid healthy.

Seventy percent of our autoimmune system is found in our intestines, which is known as GALT, or gut-associated lymphoid tissue." At the point when the digestive coating becomes aroused, it can set off an invulnerable reaction. According to research, this contributes to the onset of thyroid disease."

Suggested following a Mediterranean diet to help reduce inflammation. Dr. Gupta suggested aiming for four to five servings of vegetables and three to four servings of fruit daily, in addition to plenty of lean proteins and fatty fish, such as salmon, herring, anchovies, and mackerel. This diet typically includes:3 fruits, vegetables, beans, whole grains, fish and seafood, nuts, and seeds, and healthy oils. Dr. Gupta recommended extra-virgin olive oil, expeller-pressed organic canola oil, sunflower oil, safflower oil, coconut oil, almonds, nut butters, and avocados. sources of beneficial fats.

Avoid certain foods.
Avoid processed foods that are loaded with sugar and preservatives, dyes, or sugar- and fat-free substitutes while consuming the aforementioned foods.
Processed foods, such as trans fats, high fructose corn syrup, MSG, and refined sugar, can cause intestinal inflammation, which in turn can trigger autoimmune flare-ups." This does not only affect the thyroid; the autoimmune system can also affect other parts of the body.
Cauliflower, cabbage, kale, kohlrabi, watercress, Bok choy, and Brussels sprouts are examples of

cruciferous vegetables. ""Uncooked cruciferous veggies contain natural compounds known as goitrogens (goiter makers) that might interfere with thyroid hormone synthesis. Although they may be packed with nutrients that are good for you, such as vitamin C and folate, eating a lot of raw cruciferous vegetables could harm your thyroid.

However, there is good news for those who enjoy these kinds of vegetables: You can still consume these foods for their valuable antioxidant and cancer-protective effects because the goitrogens in them are inactivated by cooking or even light steaming," Dr. Gupta added.

Consider Supplements—After Talking to a Healthcare Provider

After speaking with a healthcare professional, think about taking supplements. You may have heard that iodine, which is necessary for the synthesis of thyroid hormones, is linked to healthy thyroid function.

One of the causes of an enlarged thyroid gland and hypothyroidism worldwide is iodine deficiency." However, due to the addition of iodine to table salt and certain foods like bread and dairy, iodine deficiency is uncommon in developed nations."

To put it another way, your diet probably already contains enough iodine. Because hyperthyroidism can be caused by too much iodine, I did not recommend taking iodine pills without consulting a doctor.

On the other hand, if you think your thyroid needs more support, talk to your doctor about taking vitamin D or selenium, which have both been linked to better thyroid health.

Clinical research shows that taking 200 mcg of the mineral selenium daily can reduce anti-thyroid antibodies." You could also consume one to two Brazil nuts each day to get the mineral.

"Severe deficiency of vitamin D may be associated with autoimmune disease," states one study on vitamin D, "have your physician check your vitamin D levels and advise you about supplementation if the level is below normal I also recommended taking probiotics, which offer a whole host of health benefits." It is recommended to look for over-the-counter blends that contain the active cultures Saccharomyces boulardii and Lactobacillus acidophilus or to consume natural sources like yogurt and kefir because probiotics can help modulate the immune system, increase gut motility, and improve intestinal permeability.


**Try Your Best To Avoid These Environmental Toxins**

Endocrine disruptors—chemicals that disrupt your body's endocrine system—may cause endocrine problems in humans if they are exposed for an extended period of time.

Per fluorinated chemicals (PFCs) are one to be aware of. PFCs are made-up chemicals that repel oil and water. PFCs have been linked to thyroid disease in previous PLOS ONE studies, and these chemicals can be found in things like: some carpets, waterproof clothing, firefighting foams, non-stick cookware, leather products, and so on. In addition, exposure to phthalates (which are found in soft plastics and fragranced products) and bisphenol A (which are found in some hard plastics and canned food linings, despite the fact that many manufacturers are removing them) may disrupt thyroid hormone levels. I also advised against using antibacterial soaps that contain triclosan. Although it would be impossible to completely avoid these, the key is to reduce your exposure as much as possible, especially if you are pregnant or have little ones in the house—developing fetuses, infants, and children are more susceptible to any effects of environmental chemicals. Triclosan is an ingredient that has altered hormone regulation in animal studies (human studies are still ongoing).

It's helpful to follow some general guidelines. Instead, just wash your hands with soap and water, "Dr. Gupta stated. When you need a fragrance, use essential oils."

You can also avoid toxins by eating more fresh or frozen foods rather than canned ones, storing food in porcelain or glass instead of plastic, and keeping your home well-ventilated.

## Natural Treatments for Hypothyroidism

Thyroid hormone replacement therapy is the most common treatment for hypothyroidism. Naturally, medications frequently have side effects, and forgetting to take a pill may result in additional symptoms.

## Natural Remedies for Hypothyroidism

Alternative or natural treatments The goal of natural or alternative treatments is to address the underlying issue with the thyroid. Occasionally, thyroid issues begin as a result of:

poor diet
Stress from a poor diet and a lack of nutrients in your body are two ways to treat your thyroid condition. You can also take an herbal supplement and change your diet. Compared to taking thyroid medication, these alternatives may have fewer side effects.
People who aren't responding well to medications may also benefit from taking an herbal supplement to treat a low or underactive thyroid.
Take into consideration the five natural treatments listed below as alternatives or additions to your treatment plan.

 Selenium
Selenium According to the Trusted Source of the National Institutes of Health (NIH), selenium is a trace element that is involved in the metabolism of thyroid hormone.

Many foods contain selenium, including:
grass-fed beef
tuna

turkey and Brazil nuts Hashimoto's thyroiditis, an immune system attack on the thyroid, frequently depletes the body's supply of selenium. Some people's thyroxine, or T4, levels can be balanced by taking this trace element supplement.

Since everyone is different, it's important to talk to your doctor about how much selenium might be right for you.

Sugar-free

Diet Sugar and processed foods can cause more inflammation in the body.

T4's conversion to triiodothyronine, or T3, a different thyroid hormone, can be slowed down by inflammation. Your symptoms and thyroid disease may get worse as a result.

Additionally, eliminating sugar from your diet may help regulate your energy levels because it only provides a short-term energy boost. Also, eliminating sugar from your eating regimen might help your feelings of anxiety and skin.

Adopting a sugar-free diet can be difficult, but the benefits to your thyroid health may be worth it.

Vitamin B

Consuming particular vitamin supplements can have an effect on the health of your thyroid.

Vitamin B-12 levels can be affected by low thyroid hormone levels. You might be able to repair some of the damage that hypothyroidism caused by taking a vitamin B-12 supplement.

Thyroid disease can make people tired, but vitamin B-12 can help. Your levels of vitamin B-1 are also impacted by the illness. The meals listed below can help you receive extra B vitamins:

Asparagus
 peas, beans
 sesame seeds
 tuna cheese,L

Eggs, and milk all contain the recommended amount of vitamin B12. Find out from your doctor how much vitamin B-12 you should take.

Probiotics The NIH investigated the connection between small intestine issues and hypothyroidism.

It was discovered that hypothyroidism-associated altered gastrointestinal (GI) motility can result in SIBO—small intestinal bacterial overgrowth—and, ultimately, chronic GI symptoms like diarrhea.

Live beneficial bacteria in probiotic supplements can support healthy intestines and stomachs.

In addition to supplements, fermented foods and beverages like yogurt, kefir, kombucha, and some cheeses contain beneficial probiotics.

Probiotics, on the other hand, have not been approved for use in the treatment or prevention of any disease by the Food and Drug Administration. Check with your doctor to see if taking these supplements would be beneficial.


Diet free of gluten

For many hypothyroid patients, following a gluten-free diet is more than just a trend.

The National Foundation for Celiac Awareness claims that celiac disease affects a significant number of people who also have thyroid disease.

Gluten causes an immune response in the small intestines, causing celiac disease, a digestive disorder.

Currently, research does not support a gluten-free diet for treating thyroid disease.

However, cutting out wheat and other foods with gluten in them can help a lot of people with hypothyroidism and Hashimoto's thyroiditis feel better.

Going gluten-free has some drawbacks, though. First of all, buying gluten-free foods frequently comes at a much higher price than buying wheat-based foods.

Additionally, not all gluten-free prepackaged foods are healthy. This is due to the fact that these foods may contain more fat and less fiber than wheat-containing products.

Bonus

For many, natural thyroid treatment has more advantages than disadvantages.

However, a natural thyroid treatment plan is not appropriate for you if you have had surgery to remove your thyroid. Before beginning any treatment, you should, as always, talk to your doctor about your options.

# Chapter Six

# Children's thyroid illness

Children's thyroid disease Despite the fact that children have thyroid disease less frequently than adults do, the signs and symptoms can be similar. However, there are a few significant distinctions that need to be made clear.

The thyroid gland is just below the Adam's apple in the front of the neck. It has an impact on each and every organ, cell, and tissue in our body and controls the rate of all chemical and metabolic processes. As a result, life and growth are dependent on the thyroid gland.

As a result, disorders of the thyroid gland have a significant impact on the human body.

At the point when the thyroid organ delivers an excess of thyroid chemical (overactive), the condition is called hyperthyroidism. At the point when the thyroid organ creates too minimal thyroid chemical (underactive), the condition is called hypothyroidism.

**Congenital hypothyroidism**

A pediatric endocrinologist or a pediatrician working with a pediatric endocrinologist typically manages thyroid conditions in children.

Hypothyroidism in the womb Hypothyroidism in the womb is a condition that affects newborns and affects about 1 in 4000 live-born babies. Due to the abnormal development of the thyroid gland, it is characterized by loss of thyroid function. The gland may be completely absent in some instances. A defect in an enzyme that results in hormone deficiency, iodine deficiency, and an abnormal pituitary gland in the brain account for about 10% of cases. Congenital hypothyroidism can result in severe mental retardation (cretinism) and growth and developmental defects if the diagnosis is delayed and prompt treatment is not provided.

Hyperthyroidism in newborns

Fortunately, newborns must undergo routine thyroid function testing since 1976. A heel prick is used to measure an infant's thyroid hormone level in the first week of life. A second blood sample is taken if any abnormalities are discovered. Thyroid hormone replacement therapy (T4 — thyroxine) is administered to the infant right away if this demonstrates congenital hypothyroidism. Typical development and advancement ought to then proceed, with no antagonistic consequences for the youngster's intellectual ability.

This condition was often overlooked prior to the introduction of newborn thyroid screening. Even after a few days, subtle signs like poor eating, constipation, a low body temperature, cool skin, a slow pulse, prolonged jaundice, more sleepiness, and less crying would show up. Other physical symptoms like dry skin and hair, poor muscle tone, slow tendon reflexes, hoarse crying, an enlarged

tongue, an umbilical hernia, and puffiness or swelling would show up after a few weeks. There would already be some devastating effects by this point. The majority of the physical symptoms would have been resolved with thyroid hormone replacement therapy, but the child would most likely have sustained permanent brain damage.
Neonatal hyperthyroidism is a rare condition characterized by an overactive thyroid gland. Neonatal hyperthyroidism is the term used to describe this condition.

Thyroid-stimulating antibodies in the mother's blood can cross the placenta and stimulate the thyroid gland of the unborn child, resulting in excessive production of thyroid hormone. The risk of an affected infant can be predicted using these stimulating antibodies, which can be measured. If antibodies are low, some newborns may not be affected at all. Because the mother's antibodies will soon be eliminated from the baby's bloodstream, typically within two to three months, treatment may not be necessary.

However, it is possible to develop severe thyrotoxicosis if the levels of stimulating antibodies are high enough in certain circumstances. The hormone imbalance will be rectified immediately with antithyroid medication.

Babies with cutting edge hyperthyroidism might show comparative side effects to those in grown-ups, like a very quick heartbeat, crabbiness, flushed wet skin, and a voracious craving with inability to flourish (for example the newborn child's body will in general be long and slender).

Fortunately, until the stimulating antibodies are eliminated from the baby's bloodstream, treatment with antithyroid medications, which are both safe and effective, will only be required for a short time. The diagnosis may be delayed by approximately a week until the infant is free of the antithyroid medication if the mother is taking a high dose of the medication. Prior to giving birth, it is recommended to work with a pediatric endocrinologist.

An autoimmune condition known as Hashimoto's thyroiditis is the most common cause of hypothyroidism in children and adolescents. The immune system of the body attacks the thyroid gland and prevents it from making thyroid hormones. This condition can begin at any age, and because the symptoms of hypothyroidism develop very slowly, the diagnosis may go unnoticed for years. Physical and mental changes will become more apparent as the thyroid gland becomes less active.

Typically, the child's unexpectedly slow growth rate and delayed skeletal development are the first signs. Because the thyroid gland becomes inflamed, the child may also have an obvious neck swelling known as a goitre. Other signs and symptoms include unusual tiredness or lethargy, dry, irritated skin, increased sensitivity to cold, weight gain or widespread swelling, poor concentration, diminished energy, and constipation.

A straightforward blood test is performed to determine the levels of thyroid hormone and thyroid stimulating hormone (TSH) in the blood if hypothyroidism is suspected. The presence of anti-thyroperoxidase and anti-thyroglobulin antibodies against the thyroid can also be helpful in confirming the diagnosis.

Children's Symptoms of Thyroid Disease Although thyroid disease typically strikes adults, it can also strike infants, young children, and adolescents. Many of the signs and symptoms of thyroid disease in children—such as changes in appetite, sleep patterns, emotions, and energy levels—are also part of normal development during this time.

Frequent Symptoms If you're concerned that there might be a problem, taking a look at some of the most common symptoms of hypothyroidism and hyperthyroidism can help you figure out what to do next.

Hashimoto's thyroiditis

The most common cause of hypothyroidism is a lack of thyroid hormone production by the thyroid gland, either because it is unable to do so (primary hypothyroidism) or because it is not being stimulated appropriately (secondary hypothyroidism).

Children with hypothyroidism may exhibit the following signs and symptoms:1 short stature or slow growth, rough, dry skin, constipation, intolerance to cold, fatigue, decreased energy, increased sleepiness, bruising easily, bone fractures, or delayed bone age on X-ray, delayed puberty. If you are concerned about your child's thyroid because they are overweight, it may be helpful to know that children who experience weight gain as a result of thyroid problems are typically shorter than was anticipated for their

Thyroid overactivity or overstimulation leads to hyperthyroidism, which is characterized by an excess of thyroid hormones.

Exophthalmos (protruding eyes) (protruding eyes) Upper eyelid droop sporadic blinking Skin that has been washed Sweating excessively Muscle fatigue Palpitation and tachycardia (rapid heartbeat) (a sense that you can feel your heart beating) High blood pressure pressure Thyroid Disease and Endocrine Dysfunction The thyroid gland is an endocrine gland.3 Emotional lability, crying easily, irritability, or excitability Short attention span Tremors Increased appetite Weight loss Other endocrine conditions like diabetes, pituitary tumors, and adrenal tumors can occur alongside thyroid disease. In a similar vein, if your child suffers from any other endocrine condition, he or she will most likely undergo testing for thyroid disease.

**Symptoms of Thyroid Disease in Children**
Thyroid disease can affect young children, adolescents, and adults as well as infants and children. Many of the signs and symptoms of thyroid disease in children—such as changes in appetite, sleep patterns, emotions, and energy

levels—are also part of normal development during this time.

**Frequent Symptoms**

If you're concerned that there might be a problem, taking a look at some of the most common symptoms of hypothyroidism and hyperthyroidism can help you figure out what to do next.

Hypothyroidism

The most common cause of hypothyroidism is a lack of thyroid hormone production by the thyroid gland, either because it is unable to do so (primary hypothyroidism) or because it is not being stimulated appropriately (secondary hypothyroidism).

**The following signs and symptoms**

emotional instability, the tendency to cry easily, irritability, or excitement
limited ability to focus
Tremors
higher appetite
Loss of weight
thyroid gland that is larger (goiter)
Exophthalmos (protruding eyes) (protruding eyes)

lax upper eyelids

sporadic blinking

blotchy skin

excessive perspiration

muscle tremor

palpitations and tachycardia (rapid heartbeat) (a sense that you can feel your heart beating)

elevated blood pressureIf you are concerned about your child's thyroid because they are overweight, it may be helpful to know that children who experience weight gain as a result of thyroid problems are typically shorter than was anticipated for their.

Thyroid overactivity or overstimulation leads to hyperthyroidism, which is characterized by an excess of thyroid hormones.

Exophthalmos (protruding eyes) Upper eyelid lag Infrequent blinking Flushed skin Excessive sweating Muscle weakness Tachycardia (rapid heartbeat) and palpitation (a sense that you can feel your heart beating) High blood pressure

**Thyroid Disease and Endocrine Dysfunction**

The thyroid gland is an endocrine gland. Emotional lability, crying easily, irritability, or excitability Short attention span Tremors Increased appetite

Weight loss Other endocrine conditions like diabetes, pituitary tumors, and adrenal tumors can occur alongside thyroid disease. In a similar vein, if your child suffers from any other endocrine condition, he or she will most likely undergo testing for thyroid disease.


Complications

Thyroid disease can cause developmental issues in children, especially if it is not treated.1 Children with noncancerous thyroid disease may also be more likely to develop certain types of thyroid cancer.

Thyroid disease can cause the following problems in children:

Slow progress:
 If thyroid disease is not treated before adolescence, children may not grow to their full potential.

Premature puberty:
Myxedema: In boys and girls, delayed puberty can be reflected in delayed menstruation and sluggish sexual development1. Myxedema, or skin swelling,

is a condition that can be brought on by severe hypothyroidism.

Issues with fertility:
Thyroid disease can cause infertility in later life in both boys and girls. Heart problems can also occur during pregnancy and delivery for women who become pregnant. Chronic thyroid issues are linked to high blood pressure, heart failure, and arrhythmias (irregular heartbeats).

Cancer:
Children with HT may develop thyroid cancer. Fortunately, children with thyroid disease have a favorable prognosis. The complications can seem concerning to parents of thyroid disease patients. Thyroid disease can be a lifelong condition, but with the right treatment and consistent management of thyroid hormone levels, these complications can be avoided.

When to See a Doctor
When to See a Doctor If your family has a history of thyroid problems, you should talk to your pediatrician about how often your child should have thyroid disease screening tests.

Make an appointment with a doctor if you notice that they have symptoms of hyperthyroidism or hypothyroidism so that the cause can be determined and treated.

Thyroid hormone levels will likely be measured in your child's blood by the doctor. Children with hypothyroidism may have low levels of free thyroxine (free T4) and high levels of thyroid stimulating hormone (TSH).8 Children with hyperthyroidism typically have high levels of T4 and and triiodothyronine (T3), as well as low TSH levels

In order to rule out any other conditions, she may also order imaging studies or diagnostic tests.

Hypothyroidism in Children

Children with hypothyroidism The thyroid is a crucial gland, and problems with it may be more common than you think: Thyroid disease affects more than 12% of Americans over the course of their lives. Children and newborns alike can be affected by this disease at any age.

Hypothyroidism in Children A family history of the condition is the most common cause of hypothyroidism in children. Thyroid disease is more likely to affect children whose parents, grandparents, or siblings have hypothyroidism. This is also true if there is a history of thyroid-related immune issues in the family.

During puberty, autoimmune conditions like Graves' disease and Hashimoto's thyroiditis are more common. Girls are more likely than boys to be affected by these thyroid conditions.

Other common causes of children's hypothyroidism include:

Insufficient iodine
in a youngster's eating routine
being brought into the world with a nonfunctional thyroid or
without a thyroid organ (likewise called inherent hypothyroidism)
inappropriate treatment of a mother's thyroid infection
during pregnancy
strange pituitary organ
Side effects of Hypothyroidism in Youngsters
Babies
Hypothyroidism happens at whatever stage in life, however the side effects differ in kids. Symptoms begin in the first few weeks or months after birth in

newborns. Parents and doctors may not notice the symptoms because they are so subtle.

**Symptoms of Hypothyroidism in Children**
**Newborns**
yellowing of the skin and whites of the eyes
constipation
poor feeding
cold skin
decreased crying
loud breathing
sleeping more often/decreased activity
larger soft spot on the head
A large tongue

Toddlers and Gradeschoolers
The issues associated with hypothyroidism that begin in infancy can be different for each age group. Symptoms of thyroid problems in young children include:
limbs and height that are shorter than average
slower mental development later development of permanent teeth later onset of puberty
heart rate that is slower than usual hair that is brittle and puffy facial features

The following are the most typical adult thyroid symptoms that kids experience:

fatigue, diarrhea, and dry skin

Teens

Teens have dry skin, constipation, and tiredness. Teen hypothyroidism is more common in girls than in boys, and it is usually caused by the autoimmune disease Hashimoto's thyroiditis. Teenagers who have a family history of autoimmune diseases like Graves' disease, Hashimoto's thyroiditis, or type 1 diabetes are more likely to get thyroid disease. Thyroid disease is also more common in children with genetic disorders like Down syndrome.

**Symptoms In Teenagers**

Teenage symptoms are similar to those of adults. However, the signs and symptoms may be difficult to identify. The following physical symptoms are frequently experienced by adolescents with hypothyroidism:

Gaining weight slowed growth

Being shorter in height makes one look younger than their actual age. Slow breast development later starts.

Irregular or heavy menstrual bleeding

Delayed puberty in boys with larger testicles
Arid skin
Fragile nails and hair
Constipation
Swollen face
Hoarse voice
Enlarged thyroid gland
Stiffness and pain in the muscles and joints
Teenagers with hypothyroidism may also experience less obvious behavioral changes. These signs Incorporate
tiredness
forgetfulness
issues with behavior or mood
Issues with academic performance
depression difficulty focusing

Diagnosis and Treatment of Hypothyroidism in Children
Levothyroxine (Synthroid), a medication, is typically used as daily thyroid hormone therapy.
The dosage will be determined by your doctor based on a variety of factors, including your child's age.

Treatment

Treatment for an infant with thyroid illness is more fruitful when begun inside the youngster's most memorable month of life. Low thyroid hormone levels can result in problems with the nervous system or delays in development if they are not treated. However, these issues rarely occur because babies are routinely screened by doctors within the first four weeks of their lives.

Bonus

Low thyroid function is a common issue that can be easily diagnosed and treated. The treatment for hypothyroidism is long lasting, however your kid will carry on with an ordinary existence

**How do you care for your child at home Against Thyroid Disease**

Make sure your child takes his or her medication for thyroid hormones at the same time each day. The majority of physicians advise taking it 30 minutes before breakfast. It should not be taken with iron, calcium, or vitamin pills by your child.

Make sure your child goes to the doctor at least once or twice a year. Regular blood tests will be required of your child. He or she is ensured to be receiving the appropriate amount of thyroid hormone through these tests.

Ensure that your child consumes a calcium-rich, healthy diet. Milk, yogurt, cheese, and dark green vegetables are sources of calcium.

**How To Stop Children From Developing Hypothyroidism**

Your child needs to take a thyroid hormone pill every day. A blood test should also be administered to your child at least once a year. This ensures that the patient is taking the appropriate dosage of medication. Your child will continue to take medication to make up for the hormone the thyroid gland doesn't make.

Hypothyroidism is a potentially fatal condition. However, following treatment, children typically thrive. The majority of parents notice that their children perform better in school and have more energy as a result of treatment. Children also resume normal growth.

A crucial component of your child's treatment and safety is follow-up care. Make and keep all appointments, and ask your doctor or nurse for advice by calling. if your child is struggling. In addition, it's a good idea to keep track of your child's medications and test results.

# Chapter Seven

# Diet and supplements for a healthy Thyroid

The diet and thyroid disorders information in

The factsheet Thyroid and diet is also available in Polish.
There aren't any particular foods or supplements that can help treat thyroid problems.

It's important to eat a variety of foods in the right amounts to keep your health as good as it can be. suggests that you try to:

Choose unsaturated oils and spreads in minimal amounts. consume plenty of fluids (at least 6 to 8 glasses a day) It is not always simple to keep up. a varied and healthy diet, and as a result, some people may wish to take additional vitamins and supplements. base meals on higher fiber starchy foods like potatoes, bread, rice, or pasta have some dairy or dairy alternatives eat some beans, pulses, fish, eggs, meat, and other protein choose unsaturated oils and spreads, and You should avoid taking too many vitamins and supplements if you decide to take them. This is due to the fact that some can affect your thyroid function or the results of your thyroid blood test.

Before beginning any vitamin or supplement regimen, it is highly recommended that you seek the appropriate guidance from your pharmacist or physician.

Vitamin D

Vitamin D is necessary for healthy bones, teeth, and muscles and helps regulate the production of calcium and phosphate. Some vitamin D levels may also have thyroid problems, but the connection isn't clear and could just be a coincidence.

The National Health Service (NHS) recommends that all adults and children over the age of five take a supplement containing 10 milligrams of vitamin D per day due to the possibility that the majority of people are deficient in the vitamin—especially in the autumn and winter, when there is less sunlight in the UK. This is true for the majority of people during the fall and winter, but you should be concerned that you won't get enough sunlight at other times of the year, such as when you don't go outside often or when you usually cover yourself with clothes.
Consider taking 10 mg of vitamin D supplements throughout the year if you have dark skin because you run the risk of not getting enough vitamin D from sunlight.

Calcium
A few calcium-rich foods and supplements hinder the absorption of levothyroxine. To ensure that there is no significant change in blood thyroxine levels, there should be a gap of four hours between the two. Even though it has less fat, semi-skimmed or

skimmed milk still has a lot of calcium, even if you're trying to lose weight.

Lodine
Iodine, which is necessary for the production of thyroxine, is essential for people who have a healthy thyroid. Because it is necessary to ensure the development of a baby's brain during pregnancy and early life, it is especially important for pregnant women.

Iodine supplements are not necessary if you are taking levothyroxine to treat hypothyroidism (an underactive thyroid) or a goitre (thyroid swelling).

Iodine supplements are unnecessary and can make hyperthyroidism (overactive thyroid) worse if you are receiving treatment for it. The benefits of the anti-thyroid medications may be diminished by the additional iodine.

Soya
Soya prevents thyroxine from being absorbed, people who take thyroxine should try to avoid soy. If you want to take thyroxine while eating soy, you should wait as long as possible before taking the soy.

There is evidence that authorities in countries like Ireland, Australia, New Zealand, and Japan stopped selling certain brands of soya milk because they contained excessive amounts of iodine or were heavily enriched with seaweed products that naturally contain iodine.

## Kelp

Avoid products like kelp because they may affect thyroid health and function. Seaweed is the source of kelp, which is naturally high in iodine. Because of this, it is sometimes sold as a "thyroid booster" and comes in tablets and dry forms. Thyroid disease sufferers receive no health benefits from it, just as they do from iodine itself.

## Iron Tablets

Some medications, like iron tablets (ferrous sulfate), can make it harder for thyroxine to be absorbed. Thyroxine and iron should be taken four hours apart, according to some medical professionals. Follow your doctor's or pharmacist's instructions. Keep in mind that some tablets for multivitamins contain iron.

## Brassicas

Brassicas In some cases, cabbage, cauliflower, kale, and other brassicas may contribute to the development of a goitre, which is a swelling or enlargement of the thyroid gland. However, consumption of these vegetables would need to be extremely high before this becomes a real concern. This typically is not a problem and the risk is very low in the UK, where normal dietary practices are followed.

## Selenium

Selenium is thought to aid in thyroid function and can be found in Brazil nuts, tuna, sardines, eggs, and legumes like beans, chickpeas, and lentils. All of these are foods that should be included in a healthy, well-balanced diet. Because too much selenium can be harmful to health, you should not take selenium supplements until your natural levels have been measured.

Selenium is also suggested for people with mild thyroid eye disease as a treatment.

## Zinc

Zinc is thought to aid in thyroid function and can be found in shellfish, beef, chicken, and legumes like beans, chickpeas, and lentils. All of these are foods that should be included in a healthy, well-balanced diet.

Always take the recommended dose, even though it's tempting to believe that taking large amounts of some supplements will benefit us, exceeding the RI can frequently cause us more harm than good. We advise you not to take any vitamins or supplements in large quantities, and please remember to check the patient information leaflet for your thyroid medication to see if taking supplements is contraindicated. Unless otherwise directed, you should always take them at least four hours apart from your thyroid medication to prevent problems with absorption.

Please consult your physician or pharmacist if you have any questions about whether you should take vitamins or other supplements.

**Which diet is best for hypothyroidism?**
When you have an underactive thyroid, especially if you take medication for it, it's important to watch what you eat.

metabolism is slowed down by an underactive thyroid. The condition can result in mild weight gain of 5 to 10 pounds and bloating. The medication levothyroxine has the potential to aid in the regulation of thyroid hormone levels and alleviate symptoms such as weight gain.

The well-established pattern of consuming fewer calories at meals and burning more calories during physical activity continues when hormone levels are controlled.

Despite the fact that there are some useful tips for maintaining key nutrients and avoiding drug interactions, the ideal diet for people with hypothyroidism will look very much like a healthy diet for anyone.

Eat a variety of fruits and vegetables because they are the best way to get nutrients into your body. Consuming at least five portions each day will ensure that you get the most of these necessary vitamins and minerals. Consult a doctor before taking any additional vitamins or supplements.

**Important Nutrients to Watch for in Hypothyroidism**

Calcium

Consuming foods high in calcium can prevent levothyroxine, a synthetic hormone used to treat hypothyroidism, from being absorbed. Chewable antacids, for example, may contain calcium.

Levothyroxine should generally be taken without food because of the effects of calcium. Gel and liquid forms are known to reduce interactions with calcium and other nutrients in the event that this causes stomach upset.

Fiber

Synthetic thyroid hormones, such as levothyroxine, have been shown to be less effective when supplemented with excessive amounts of fiber. Fiber supplements are generally not advised if you eat fruit and vegetables as part of a healthy diet.

Iodine

A healthy thyroid and the production of the hormone thyroxine are dependent on iodine. If you have hypothyroidism and take levothyroxine, a synthetic version of thyroxine, you don't need to take iodine supplements. However, taking iodine can exacerbate symptoms of hyperthyroidism, or an overactive thyroid. Your doctor can help you determine how much dietary iodine you need to meet your needs if you have hypothyroidism as a result of an iodine deficiency.

Iron

Another mineral that can make levothyroxine less effective is iron. Before increasing your iron intake, consult your doctor. Levothyroxine should be taken at least two hours before or after taking any iron supplements, including iron-containing multivitamins.

Seaweed and kelp

Kelp has naturally high levels of iodine, so people with hypothyroidism should avoid it.

Selenium

which can be found in sardines, tuna, beans, Brazil nuts, eggs, and other foods, has also been linked to better thyroid health. However, a lot of selenium is definitely not something to be thankful for, thus supplements are not suggested.

Soy

Another food that can prevent levothyroxine from being absorbed is soy. Again, taking the hormone a few hours before or after eating soy is best. Check the labels of the soy milk you buy to see if it contains iodine.

Vitamin D

It has been known for a long time that vitamin D helps regulate calcium and phosphorus to maintain healthy teeth and bones. However, more recent research has shown that endocrine conditions like diabetes, hypothyroidism, and Hashimoto's disease may also be influenced by vitamin D.

Due to the prevalence of vitamin deficiency, there may be a coincidental link between hypothyroidism and low vitamin D levels in some studies.

Zinc

According to the British Thyroid Foundation, zinc Zinc is another mineral that is thought to be beneficial to thyroid health. It can be found in legumes (beans), beef, chicken, and shellfish, and preliminary studies have suggested that vitamin D supplements may be beneficial for thyroid conditions. However, more thorough research on safety and efficacy is required, according to the British Thyroid Foundation.

Before taking any supplements, always consult a doctor or pharmacist because it is best to get vitamins and minerals from food. It can be harmful to take more vitamins than recommended, which can result in inaccurate thyroid blood tests. In addition, if you are taking any medication for hypothyroidism, make sure to read the package insert to see if there are any side effects.

**Foods to Avoid While Taking Levothyroxine**
The synthetic hormone levothyroxine is frequently prescribed to people who have hypothyroidism. Although any undesirable interactions can generally be avoided by timing and method of intake, there are a number of foods and beverages that can reduce the effectiveness of the medication.

Levothyroxine may not be as well absorbed when consumed with iron-, calcium-, and fiber-rich foods, according to some research. To avoid poor absorption, take calcium, iron, or fiber supplements at least four hours after taking levothyroxine.

Levothyroxine tablets should generally be taken without food 30 to 60 minutes before or after drinking coffee or other caffeinated beverages.

If you take levothyroxine in a gel or liquid form rather than as a tablet, it may also have less of an effect on interactions with foods and beverages.

A sample meal plan

Typical Meal Plan

Here are some meal suggestions from the National Institutes of Health for a day with about 1,600 calories.

Breakfast
a single whole wheat slice of bread

two jam teaspoons

12 cup of cereal with shredded wheat

one cup of nonfat milk

Banana

either coffee or juice

500 calories or so total for the meal.

Or:

two pieces of whole-wheat toast

two jam teaspoons

two fried eggs (using egg whites or egg substitute)

fruit juice

Banana

400 calories or so total for the meal.

Sandwich of turkey (2 oz.)

For lunch with:

1 cheese slice

2 pieces of whole grain bread

Lettuce

Tomato

Low-calorie mayonnaise, 2 teaspoons

1 small apple

400 calories or so total for the meal.

Dinner: 3 oz. of salmon cooked in 1 tablespoon of olive oil.

potato baked in 1 teaspoon of margarine

1 cup of carrots and green beans with margarine

wheat-based dinner roll

Water, iced tea, or milk.

MEAL CALORIES: Approximately 700

# Conclusion

Your thyroid is a tiny, butterfly-shaped gland located at the front of your neck. It generates hormones that control how much energy the body uses. These hormones have an impact on almost every organ in your body and regulate a number of its most crucial processes. For instance, they affect your digestion, breathing, weight, heart rate, and mood.

When you have thyroid illness, your thyroid either produces too many or too little hormones. Some of the various thyroid conditions include the following: thyroid nodules, thyroid lumps, thyroiditis, and thyroid swelling A goiter is an enlarged thyroid gland. When your thyroid gland produces more thyroid hormones than your body requires, hyperthyroidism develops. When you have hypothyroidism, your Thyroid hormone production is insufficient. Thyrotoxic cancer lumps in the thyroid gland and thyroid nodules In some circumstances, your healthcare provider might also do a biopsy.

The type of issue, its seriousness, and your symptoms all influence the appropriate course of treatment. Treatment options include medicine, radioiodine therapy, and thyroid surgery.